KIDNEY STONES DIET

Guide On   Eating A Healthy
Diet And Improve Your Health

Gillian C. Wheeler

Table of Contents

CHAPTER1

What are Kidney stones

Kidney stones are a typical infirmity that influences a huge number of individuals consistently. They are hard mineral deposits that can cause severe pain and discomfort and form inside the kidneys. Kidney stones can be brought on by a variety of factors, including dehydration, genetics, and diet, and can be as small as grains or as large as rocks. They commonly structure when the pee becomes concentrated, permitting minerals and different substances to take shape and structure strong masses.

The side effects of kidney stones can fluctuate contingent upon the size and area of the stone. Certain individuals might encounter no side effects by any means, while others might encounter serious torment toward the back or midsection, queasiness, spewing, and trouble peeing. During routine medical examinations or imaging tests, kidney stones may be detected in some instances. Larger stones may necessitate medical intervention, such as surgery or shock wave lithotripsy, while the majority of kidney stones will pass naturally without treatment.

The best way to avoid kidney stones is to prevent them. Your risk of developing kidney stones can be reduced by drinking a lot of water, eating a healthy diet, and avoiding too much sodium and animal protein. On the off chance that you in all actuality do encounter side effects of kidney stones, it is critical to look for clinical consideration immediately to forestall confusions and guarantee appropriate treatment. With the right consideration and consideration, the vast majority can recuperate from kidney stones and proceed to have solid, dynamic existences.

From the minerals and salts in the urine, kidney stones are small, hard deposits. Ordinarily, these stones are comprised of calcium oxalate and are about the size of a grain of sand, yet they can develop bigger over the long haul. When they attempt to pass through the urinary tract, they can cause severe pain and discomfort.

CHAPTER2

What are the reasons for kidney stones

The reasons for kidney stones can shift, however most normally, they are the aftereffect of parchedness or an irregularity of specific minerals in the pee. Minerals that stick together to form a stone are more likely to stick together if the person is dehydrated, which can make the urine more concentrated. Additionally, kidney stones may be exacerbated by a diet high in animal protein, sugar, and salt. Kidney stones can also be made more likely by certain medical conditions like hyperparathyroidism, gout, and chronic kidney disease.

Way of life elements can likewise assume a part in the development of kidney stones. The development of stones may be exacerbated by a decreased urine flow caused by inactivity. Kidney stones can also be more likely to occur in people who are overweight or obese. Hereditary qualities may likewise assume a part, as certain individuals are more inclined to creating kidney stones than others. To avoid kidney stones and keep your kidneys in good health, it's important to know what causes them.

When minerals and salts in the urine stick together, kidney stones, also known as renal calculi, form in the kidneys. These deposits can cause a variety of symptoms and range in size from small particles to large stones. Pain in the lower back, abdomen, or groin is one of the most common signs of kidney stones. This aggravation can be extreme and may go back and forth in waves. Nausea and vomiting, frequent urination, and blood in the urine are additional signs of kidney stones.

The majority of the time, the movement of kidney stones into the ureters, which are the tubes that connect the kidneys to the bladder, is what causes the symptoms of kidney stones. As the stones travel through the ureters, they can cause blockages and bothering, which can prompt torment and different side effects. The size and position of the stones can affect how severe the symptoms are. While larger stones may necessitate medical intervention to be removed, smaller stones can pass through the urinary tract without causing any symptoms.

It is essential to seek medical attention if you experience symptoms of kidney stones. Your PCP can perform tests to analyze the condition and decide the best course of treatment. Painkillers and plenty of fluids can be used to help kidney stones pass through the urinary tract in some cases. In different cases, more obtrusive medicines like a medical procedure or shockwave lithotripsy might be important to eliminate the stones. You can aid in the prevention of complications and reduce discomfort associated with kidney stones by becoming aware of their symptoms and seeking prompt medical attention.

Kidney stones are little, hard stores made of minerals and salt that structure inside the kidneys. They can be of any size or shape, and passing through the urinary tract can be extremely painful. Kidney stones can be made more likely by a number of things, like being dehydrated, having a history of them in the family, and having certain medical conditions.

CHAPTER3

How to keep a sound eating routine. In Kidney stones

In any case, perhaps of the main figure forestalling kidney stones is keeping a sound eating routine.

An eating routine that is high in salt, meat, and handled food varieties can build the gamble of creating kidney stones. This is on the grounds that these kinds of food varieties can cause an expansion in the degrees of calcium, oxalate, and uric corrosive in the pee, which can add to the development of kidney stones. A diet high in fruits, vegetables, and whole grains, on the other hand, can help prevent kidney stones by reducing the amount of these minerals in the urine and providing the body with essential nutrients.

To avoid kidney stones, it is essential to consume a lot of water in addition to eating a healthy diet. Drinking sufficient water can assist with weakening the pee and diminish the convergence of minerals that can add to stone development. If you are physically active or live in a hot climate, you should drink at least 8-10 glasses of water per day. You can improve your overall health and significantly lower your risk of developing kidney stones by making these straightforward adjustments to your diet and lifestyl

Kidney stones are little, hard stores that structure in the kidneys. Minerals and salts found in urine make up their composition. These stones, which can be as small as a golf ball or a grain of sand, can be very painful to pass through the urinary tract. Among the various kinds of kidney stones are calcium, uric acid, and struvite stones. A family history of kidney stones, dehydration, a diet high in salt and protein, and certain medical conditions like gout and inflammatory bowel disease are all risk factors for kidney stones.

Drinking a lot of fluids is one of the most common treatments for kidney stones. Expanding water admission can assist with flushing out the stones and keep new ones from framing. To help ease the pain caused by passing the stones, pain medication may also be prescribed. For bigger stones, operations might be important to eliminate them. These strategies might incorporate extracorporeal shock wave lithotripsy (ESWL), which utilizations shock waves to separate the stones into more modest pieces that can be passed all the more effectively, or ureteroscopy, which includes utilizing a little extension to eliminate the stones from the urinary plot.

A diet high in certain nutrients, such as calcium, oxalate, and uric acid, is one of the main factors that contribute to the development of kidney stones. Calcium oxalate stones are the most well-known sort of kidney stone, and are shaped when there is a lot of calcium and oxalate in the pee. A diet high in purines, such as seafood and red meat, can increase the amount of uric acid in the urine, which can lead to the formation of uric acid stones. Other dietary factors that can add to kidney stone arrangement incorporate lack of hydration, high sodium admission, and low potassium consumption.

Changes to one's diet that decrease intake of calcium, oxalate, and uric acid and increase intake of hydration and potassium are essential for preventing kidney stones. This can be accomplished by sticking to a diet high in fruits, vegetables, and whole grains and avoiding foods high in oxalate, like nuts, rhubarb, and spinach. Additionally, it is essential to consume a lot of water throughout the day to maintain a diluted urine and prevent the accumulation of minerals and salts. Individuals can enjoy improved overall health and a significantly lower risk of kidney stones by making these dietary changes.

One of the main food sources to zero in on while attempting to forestall kidney stones is water. Drinking a lot of water helps make the urine less concentrated, which reduces the likelihood of kidney stones forming. In addition to drinking water, people should focus on eating foods high in citric acid. Citrus extract can assist with forestalling the development of stones by restricting to calcium in the pee and keeping it from shaping gems. Citric acid-rich fruits and vegetables include grapefruits, limes, lemons, and oranges.

Another significant nutrition type to zero in on while attempting to forestall kidney stones is calcium-rich food sources. Consuming calcium-rich foods can actually help prevent kidney stones from forming, despite the fact that this may appear counterintuitive. This is due to the fact that calcium binds with oxalates in the digestive tract, limiting the amount of oxalates that can be absorbed into the bloodstream and eliminated through urine. Food varieties that are high in calcium incorporate milk, cheddar, and yogurt.

Last but not least, individuals ought to concentrate on reducing the amount of oxalates in their diets. Oxalates are substances that can add to the arrangement of kidney stones.

Food varieties that are high in oxalates incorporate spinach, rhubarb, beets, and nuts. While it may not be important to totally dispose of these food varieties from the eating regimen, people ought to plan to devour them with some restraint.

Overall, changing one's diet can be a good way to avoid kidney stones. People can help lower their risk of developing kidney stones by focusing on drinking plenty of water, eating foods that are high in citric acid, and eating foods that are high in calcium. Moreover, diminishing the admission of food varieties that are high in oxalates can likewise be helpful. People can help improve kidney health as a whole and lower their risk of painful kidney stones by making these changes.

Kidney stones are a difficult and normal condition that can be forestalled by rolling out dietary improvements. People can reduce their risk of developing kidney stones by avoiding certain foods. One of the fundamental food sources to keep away from is high oxalate food varieties. Oxalate is a characteristic substance found in numerous food sources that can prompt the development of calcium oxalate stones. Spinach, beets, rhubarb, and nuts are all examples of foods high in oxalate.

Salt is another food that should be avoided to prevent kidney stones. Too much sodium can make the amount of calcium in the urine more concentrated, which can cause stones to form. Handled food sources, cheap food, and canned soups are high in sodium. It is suggested that people consume no more than 2,300 milligrams of sodium per day.

Salt is another food that should be avoided to prevent kidney stones. Too much sodium can make the amount of calcium in the urine more concentrated, which can cause stones to form. Handled food sources, cheap food, and canned soups are high in sodium. It is suggested that people consume no more than 2,300 milligrams of sodium per day.

Lastly, individuals should limit their intake of animal protein. Animal protein can raise the amount of uric acid in the urine, which can cause uric acid stones to form. Red meat, poultry, fish, and eggs are all examples of animal protein. It is suggested that people limit their admission of creature protein and choose plant-based protein sources like beans, lentils, and tofu all things considered.

There are a few other dietary changes that can help prevent kidney stones in addition to drinking more fluids. One significant change is to restrict the admission of specific kinds of food varieties and beverages. Oxalate-rich foods like spinach, rhubarb, and almonds can make kidney stones more likely. Drinks that are high in sugar or caffeine, like soda or coffee, can also cause kidney stones to form. To lower your risk of developing kidney stones, it's important to limit or avoid these foods and drinks.

Increasing your intake of certain nutrients is another dietary modification that can assist in the prevention of kidney stones. Calcium and magnesium, in particular, have been shown to lower the risk of kidney stones. Given that calcium is frequently present in kidney stones, this may seem counterintuitive. However, by binding to oxalate in the digestive tract and preventing its absorption into the bloodstream, calcium can actually help prevent the formation of stones. Magnesium, on the other hand, can stop crystals from growing and prevent calcium-based stones from forming. Dairy products, leafy greens, and nuts are sources of calcium and magnesium

Limiting your sodium intake is another important piece of advice for sticking to a diet that prevents kidney stones. Consuming unreasonable measures of sodium can expand how much calcium in your pee, which can add to the arrangement of kidney stones. To restrict your sodium consumption, it is prescribed to keep away from handled food varieties, canned merchandise, and cheap food, as these are much of the time high in sodium. All things considered, settle on new entire food varieties, like organic products, vegetables, and entire grains.

Generally, rolling out dietary improvements is a compelling method for forestalling the advancement of kidney stones. You can lower your risk of developing this painful condition by following these guidelines and eating a diet that prevents kidney stones. To keep your kidneys healthy and free of stones, remember to drink plenty of water, limit animal protein and foods high in oxalate, and cut back on sodium.

One more key part of a kidney stone counteraction diet is scaling back food sources that are high in oxalates. Oxalates are intensifies found in many plant-based food varieties, including spinach, beets, nuts, and chocolate, and they can add to the development of kidney stones in certain individuals. You don't have to completely avoid these foods, but you should limit your consumption and make sure you get enough calcium, which can help bind with oxalates and prevent them from forming stones. Salt, refined sugar, and animal protein are other foods to avoid or limit.

Last but not least, you might want to think about including more foods in your diet that have been shown to help prevent kidney stones. These incorporate citrus organic products, which are high in citrate, a compound that can assist with dissolving stones; mixed greens like kale and collard greens, which are low in oxalates and high in calcium; and whole grains like brown rice and quinoa, which have a lot of fiber and other nutrients that help the kidneys in general. You can make a delicious and nutritious diet for kidney stone prevention with a little planning and effort.

Limiting alcohol and caffeine intake, which can dehydrate the body and raise the risk of kidney stones, is essential in conjunction with eating a well-balanced diet. Smoking ought to be avoided as well because it has the potential to harm the kidneys and raise the risk of kidney disease. People can maintain good kidney health and avoid kidney stones by adhering to these guidelines and making mindful food choices.

A healthy diet is important for all aspects of health, including the health of the kidneys. The kidneys are responsible for removing waste and excess fluids from the body, and maintaining their health is essential to avoiding kidney stones. A diet that is high in sugar, sodium, and protein can make you more likely to get kidney stones, and a diet that doesn't give you enough of the essential nutrients can also hurt how well your kidneys work. Consequently, it is fundamental to follow a fair eating regimen to advance kidney wellbeing.

Vitamins, minerals, and antioxidants should be present in a variety of foods in a well-balanced diet for kidney stone prevention. It is fundamental to consume an eating regimen that is wealthy in organic products, vegetables, entire grains, and lean proteins. These foods supply essential nutrients that aid in the prevention of kidney stones and support kidney function. Additionally, sodium, animal proteins, and refined sugars, which can raise the risk of kidney stones, must be avoided at all costs.

In conclusion, avoiding kidney stones requires eating a well-balanced diet. Whole grains, lean proteins, and a variety of fruits and vegetables are all part of a well-balanced diet that can help support kidney function and lower the risk of kidney stones. Sodium, animal proteins, and refined sugars, which can raise the risk of developing kidney stones, must also be avoided at all costs. Individuals can safeguard their kidney health and prevent the development of kidney stones by eating a well-balanced diet.

Adjusting your eating routine is fundamental for

forestalling kidney stones. You can avoid kidney stones by including a variety of foods in your diet. These food varieties give fundamental supplements to your body as well as decrease the gamble of creating kidney stones.

Water is one of the most important foods to include in your diet to prevent kidney stones. To eliminate toxins and other waste products from your body, it is essential to drink enough water. Water aids in diluting urine, lowering the likelihood of kidney stones forming. Drinking no less than 8-10 glasses of water daily is suggested. Alongside water, different liquids, for example, new natural product juices, coconut water, and home grown teas can likewise be remembered for your eating routine.

One more food to remember for your eating routine for kidney stone anticipation is calcium-rich food varieties. Calcium is not to blame for kidney stones, contrary to popular belief. In point of fact, a low-calcium diet can make it more likely that you will get kidney stones. In the intestine, calcium forms a bond with oxalate, preventing its absorption into the bloodstream. The risk of developing kidney stones is reduced as a result of this decrease in the amount of oxalate that reaches the kidneys. Food varieties like milk, cheddar, and yogurt are astounding wellsprings of calcium.

Food sources that are high in citrate content ought to likewise be remembered for your eating regimen for kidney stone anticipation. Natural inhibitor of kidney stone formation is citrate. It forestalls the collection of gems and restrains the development of stones. Citrate is abundant in citrus fruits like limes, grapefruits, oranges, and lemons. These organic products can be polished off in their regular structure or as juices. If you eat these foods, you can lower your risk of developing kidney stones.

In conclusion, maintaining a healthy diet is essential to avoiding kidney stones. Consuming foods high in citrate, calcium, and water can help lower the likelihood of kidney stones forming. A well-balanced diet that provides your body with all of the necessary nutrients is critical. Kidney stones can also be avoided with regular exercise, a healthy lifestyle, and a well-balanced diet.

CHAPTER4

**What the way of life changes
for Kidney stones**

Notwithstanding clinical medicines, way of life changes can likewise be powerful in forestalling kidney stones. A diet high in fruits and vegetables and low in salt and animal protein can help lower the risk of developing kidney stones. Alcohol and sugary drinks can also be avoided. Kidney stones can also be avoided by being physically active and maintaining a healthy weight. People who have kidney stones can manage their condition and lower their risk of developing more stones in the future by making these adjustments and adhering to a treatment plan that has been prescribed by a healthcare professional.

When they pass through the urinary tract, kidney stones, which are hardened deposits of minerals and salts, can cause severe pain. They form in the kidneys. They can be brought on by a number of things, like a diet high in certain substances, dehydration, and genetics. A kidney stone is a serious health issue to be aware of because it is estimated to affect one in ten people at some point in their lives. Fortunately, there are dietary modifications that can significantly lower the likelihood of developing kidney stones, a painful condition.

. When minerals and other substances in urine form hard crystals, kidney stones are a common, painful condition.

Changing one's diet is one of the many methods for avoiding kidney stones. By zeroing in on specific food varieties, people can assist with diminishing their gamble of creating kidney stones.

Finally, avoiding kidney stones necessitates maintaining a healthy weight. Corpulence and being overweight are risk factors for kidney stones, as they can prompt changes in pee creation and an expanded gamble of creating insulin obstruction. By keeping a solid load through a fair eating routine and ordinary activity, people can decrease their gamble of creating kidney stones.

It is essential to collaborate with a medical professional to devise a customized strategy for avoiding kidney stones that takes into account each person's requirements and medical history.

Kidney stones are a condition that affects millions of people worldwide and can be extremely painful. Luckily, it is feasible to decrease the probability of creating kidney stones by rolling out specific dietary improvements. A kidney stone prevention diet is one of the most effective ways to prevent kidney stones. The foods on this diet are low in oxalate, calcium, and sodium, all of which play a major role in the formation of kidney stones.

To keep a kidney stone counteraction diet, polishing off a lot of water over the course of the day is significant. It is possible to avoid kidney stones and flush out toxins by drinking at least 8 to 10 glasses of water per day. It is additionally prescribed to restrict the utilization of high-oxalate food varieties, like spinach, beets, rhubarb, and okra. Additionally, reducing your intake of animal protein, such as fish, meat, and poultry, can help stop kidney stones from forming.

CHAPTER5

Ingredients that can help lower the risk of stone formation,

Kidney stones can be a difficult and awkward condition to manage. Fortunately, there are recipes that people can use to assist with forestalling the arrangement of kidney stones. Ingredients that can help lower the risk of stone formation, such as foods high in citrate or water, are typically the focus of recipes for kidney stone prevention.

A watermelon smoothie is one example of a kidney stone prevention recipe. Watermelon is an incredible wellspring of water and citrulline, which can assist with forestalling the development of kidney stones. To make a watermelon smoothie, just mix watermelon lumps with ice and a sprinkle of lemon juice. You can likewise include other sound fixings, like spinach or chia seeds, to make the smoothie much more nutritious.

A quinoa salad with a citrus dressing is another recipe for preventing kidney stones. Quinoa is an extraordinary wellspring of protein, while citrus organic products are high in citrate. To make the serving of mixed greens, cook quinoa as per bundle directions and blend in with slashed vegetables, for example, cucumber and ringer pepper. For the dressing, whisk together lemon or lime juice, olive oil, and a dash of honey. Serve the quinoa salad with the dressing for a tasty and kidney-friendly meal.

Finally, people can likewise integrate kidney stone counteraction into their day to day snacks. Dried apricots or almonds, for instance, can be a great way to get more citrate into your diet. Drinking a lot of water throughout the day can also help flush the kidneys and lower the risk of developing stones. By integrating kidney stone avoidance recipes and sound propensities into one's way of life, people can decrease their gamble of encountering the uneasiness of kidney stones.

Kidney stones can be extremely uncomfortable and painful. It is, subsequently, critical to go to lengths to forestall their development. This can be accomplished in a number of ways, one of which is through diet, which entails eating foods that are made to help prevent the formation of kidney stones. Such feasts ought to be low in oxalates, which are the mixtures that structure kidney stones. Also, they ought to be high in supplements like calcium, magnesium, and citrate, which help to forestall kidney stones.

A spinach and chicken salad is one example of a meal that can help prevent kidney stones. Spinach is an extraordinary wellspring of calcium, magnesium, and citrate, all of which help to forestall kidney stone development. Additionally, chicken is an excellent source of protein, which is essential to overall health. Different fixings that can be added to this salad incorporate carrots, beets, and tomatoes, which are low in oxalates.

Another dinner that can assist with forestalling kidney stone development is a quinoa and vegetable pan fried food. Protein and fiber, both of which are important for overall health, can be found in abundance in quinoa. Besides, it is low in oxalates, settling on it an extraordinary decision for kidney stone counteraction. This meal is a great way to get all the nutrients you need while also preventing the formation of kidney stones when it is combined with vegetables like broccoli, cauliflower, and bell peppers.

A lentil soup with a lot of vegetables is a third meal that can help prevent kidney stones. Lentils are low in oxalates and a great source of protein and fiber. As a result, they are an excellent option for preventing kidney stones. This soup is a great way to get all the nutrients you need while also preventing kidney stones when it is made with lots of vegetables like carrots, celery, and onions. In addition, lentil soup is not difficult to make and can be delighted in by the entire family.

A condition that can be brought on by a variety of factors, such as genetics, diet, and lifestyle choices, kidney stones can be extremely painful. There are a number of steps that can be taken to either prevent or reduce the likelihood of developing kidney stones, although some people may require medical intervention to remove large stones. Changing one's diet to include foods that are low in oxalate, a substance that can cause stones, is one of the best ways to prevent the disease. With regards to snacks for kidney stone avoidance, there are a few choices that are both heavenly and nutritious. Snacking on fresh, low-oxalate fruits and vegetables like apples, berries, carrots, and cucumbers is a great option. In addition to being hydrating and healthy, these foods are also a good source of fiber and other essential nutrients that can help improve overall health. Include foods high in calcium in your snacks to prevent kidney stones. These foods can help bind with oxalate in the digestive system and prevent it from contributing to stone formation. A few decent wellsprings of calcium incorporate low-fat dairy items, like yogurt and cheddar, as well as verdant green vegetables like kale and spinach. Snacks that are both nutritious and friendly to kidney stones can be made from these foods by themselves or by combining them with other nutritious ingredients. In general, one important way to lower your risk of developing this painful condition is to include snacks that prevent kidney stones in your diet. By picking food sources that are low in oxalate and high in calcium, you can assist with supporting your general wellbeing and health while additionally getting a charge out of tasty and fulfilling snacks. There are many foods that can support the health and proper functioning of your kidneys, whether you prefer fresh fruits and vegetables or dairy and leafy greens.

Stones in the kidney can be extremely painful and cause

problems in daily life. Hard deposits that can clog the urinary tract are formed when minerals and other substances in the urine crystallize and stick together. Luckily, there are numerous ways of forestalling kidney stones from framing in any case, including rolling out dietary improvements. Here are a few ways to keep a kidney stone counteraction diet.

Above all else, drinking a lot of water is significant. One of the best ways to avoid kidney stones is to drink enough water because it helps to lower the concentration of minerals and other substances in the urine. Plan to drink no less than eight glasses of water each day, and the sky is the limit from there in the event that you're truly dynamic or live in a warm environment. You can likewise stir things up by drinking different liquids like home grown tea or coconut water, yet make a point to stay away from sweet or juiced drinks, which can really expand your gamble of creating kidney stones.

Kidney health is essential to overall health and the prevention of kidney stones. Dietary balancing is one of the most important ways to accomplish this. The most important phase in adjusting your eating routine is to restrict food sources that are high in salt and creature protein. Kidney stones can be caused by eating too much salt, and eating too much animal protein can make it more likely that you will get kidney disease.

Fruits and vegetables are an important part of a healthy diet because they contain essential vitamins and minerals that help the kidneys function properly. Entire grains and lean protein sources, like fish and poultry, are additionally significant. It means quite a bit to drink a lot of water to keep the kidneys hydrated and assist with forestalling the development of kidney stones.

CHAPTER6

Certain foods. To avoid   if you want to avoid developing kidney stones

Kidney stones are hard, gem like substances that can shape in the kidneys. They can be very difficult and can cause a great deal of uneasiness. One of the best ways of forestalling kidney stones is by adjusting your eating regimen. If you want to avoid developing kidney stones, you should avoid certain foods.

One of the primary food sources that you ought to keep away from is high-sodium food sources. Sodium is a mineral that is tracked down in salt and different food varieties. At the point when you consume a lot of sodium, it can prompt an expansion in pee calcium. This, thusly, can prompt the arrangement of kidney stones. A few instances of high-sodium food varieties that you ought to keep away from incorporate handled food sources, canned food sources, and pungent bites.

Animal protein is another food you shouldn't eat. Meat, poultry, fish, and dairy products all contain animal protein. Calcium levels in the urine can rise if you consume too much animal protein. This can likewise prompt the development of kidney stones. It is essential to consume animal protein in moderation if you do.

In conclusion, you ought to stay away from food varieties that are high in oxalates. Oxalates are natural substances that can be found in a wide variety of foods. Oxalates have the potential to bind with calcium in the urine and cause kidney stones if consumed in excess. A few instances of food varieties that are high in oxalates incorporate spinach, rhubarb, beets, nuts, and chocolate. While it is vital to eat a reasonable eating regimen, it is likewise critical to be aware of the food varieties that you devour to forestall kidney stones.

THE END